D0181674

Get Well Soon…
If Not Sooner

Table of Contents

Introduction

Since you're reading a book about getting well, I'll make the assumption that you're feeling under the weather. If so, this book is designed to help. Illness is never restricted to the body; it also has a way of infecting our thoughts. When the body feels sick, it's difficult to convince the mind to feel otherwise. Difficult, but not impossible.

The quality of your thoughts can either speed the healing process or delay it. Almost all physicians agree that the better your attitude, the better your prognosis. The quotations on the following pages are intended to buoy your spirits until recovery is complete.

In the process of compiling this book, I looked back upon my experiences as a doctor of clinical psychology. On countless occasions, I have been amazed by the resiliency of the human spirit, even in times of severe illness. Over the years, I have become convinced that every human being possesses a deep reservoir of strength which is available in times of trouble. The passages in this book are intended to remind you of the power that is already yours. So if you're sick and tired of feeling sick and tired, take these ideas to heart. The gems of wisdom in this book will help you get well soon — if not sooner.

1

Be Proactive

It has been said that there are only three kinds of people: those who *make* things happen, those who *let* things happen, and those who sit around and ask, "What happened?" When one doesn't feel well, it's tempting to sit back, do nothing, and wonder what happened. But there's a better strategy: taking responsibility for one's treatment.

The French essayist Alain observed, "There is a future that makes itself and a future we make. The real future is composed of both." *Your* real future exists in a state of health, and the sooner you return there, the better. You can speed the healing process by becoming an active participant in your treatment. Ultimately, it's up to you, not your doctor, to ensure that you receive the best medical care.

If your illness is a serious one, be prepared; you are beginning a spiritual journey as well as a physical one. But even if your ailment is something as benign as the common cold, your recovery should begin today. Otherwise, you might accidentally create a future you'd rather not imagine.

Healing is a matter of time, but it is sometimes a matter of opportunity.

Hippocrates

Fortune favors the bold
　　　but abandons the timid.

Latin Proverb

The man who insists upon seeing
with perfect clearness before he decides,
　　　never decides.

Henri Frédéric Amiel

The most important thing is to pick
a therapy you believe in and proceed with
　　　a positive attitude.

Bernie Siegel, M.D.

Think of thy deliverance as well as
　　　of thy danger.

Thomas Fuller

Above all, try something.

Franklin D. Roosevelt

The resolve to do whatever is necessary
is one of the first requirements for being
an exceptional patient.

Bernie Siegel, M.D.

He started to sing as he tackled the thing
that couldn't be done, and he did it.

Edgar A. Guest

Whatsoever thy hand findeth to do,
do it with thy might.

Ecclesiastes 9:10

Do what you can, with what you have,
where you are.

Theodore Roosevelt

Failure is the path of least persistence.

Old-Time Saying

Facing it — always facing it — that's the way to get through.

Joseph Conrad

Become an expert in your own condition.

Tom Ferguson, M.D.

Forewarned, forearmed; to be prepared
is half the victory.

Miguel de Cervantes

No man ever became wise by chance.

Seneca

Learning as much as possible about
your body and your illness is perhaps
the best tool to help you take charge.

Helen Garvy

The essence of knowledge is, having it,
to use it.

Confucius

Good loves to help him
who strives to help
himself.

Aeschylus

Don't make the mistake of passively accepting
a judgment you feel justified in questioning.
Remember: Doctors are human.
And they don't know everything.

Nancy Snyderman, M.D.

Exceptional patients want to be educated
and made "doctors" of their own cases.

Bernie Siegel, M.D.

Never despair, but if you do,
work on in despair.

Edmund Burke

Exceptional patients are self-reliant and seek
solutions rather than lapsing into depression.

Bernie Siegel, M.D.

Assume responsibility for the quality of your own life.

Norman Cousins

A sharing of responsibility with one's
physician is in the best interest
of both physician and patient.

Norman Cousins

Our grand business is not to see what lies
dimly at a distance but to do what lies
closely at hand.

Thomas Carlyle

Whatever you can do, or dream you can,
begin it. Boldness has genius, power,
and magic in it.

Goethe

He who has begun has half done.
Dare to be wise; begin!

Horace

We will either find a way or make one.

Hannibal

Do not weep; do not wax indignant.
Understand.

Baruch Spinoza

None will improve your lot
if you yourselves do not.

Bertolt Brecht

Imagine first that the present is past and,
second, that the past may yet be changed
and amended.

Viktor E. Frankl

Who escapes a duty avoids a gain.

Theodore Parker

The past is history. Make the present good,
and the past will take care of itself.

Knute Rockne

Nothing is so fatiguing as the eternal hanging
on of an uncompleted task.

William James

He who desires but acts not
breeds pestilence.

William Blake

You can't escape the responsibility
of tomorrow by evading it today.

Abraham Lincoln

One ought never to turn one's back on a
threatened danger and try to run away from it.

Sir Winston Churchill

Thought is the blossom; language the bud;
action the fruit.

Ralph Waldo Emerson

Think like a man of action and
act like a man of thought.

Henri Bergson

The shortest answer is doing.

George Herbert

The pessimist complains about the wind;
the optimist expects it to change;
the realist adjusts the sails.

William Arthur Ward

Call on God, but row away from the rocks.

Ralph Waldo Emerson

Act as if it were impossible to fail.

Dorthea Brande

When we do the best we can, we never know what miracles await.

Helen Keller

Most people spend more time and energy
going around problems than
trying to solve them.

Henry Ford

Doubt of whatever kind can be ended
by action alone.

Thomas Carlyle

The ultimate function of prophecy is not
to tell the future but to make it.

W. W. Nagar

If you have an illness, decide to be well.

Mike Samuels, M.D.

2

Good Spirits

Voltaire observed, "The longer we dwell on our misfortunes, the greater is their power to harm us." And so it is with sickness. Negative emotions are antithetical to good health. As Norman Cousins noted, "Nothing is more essential in the treatment of serious disease than liberating the patient from panic or foreboding."

If ill health has dampened *your* enthusiasm, it is time to find creative ways to cheer yourself up. The following quotations should help.

Mirth is God's medicine.
    Everybody ought to bathe in it.
                              Henry Ward Beecher

A merry heart doeth good like a medicine:
    but a broken spirit drieth the bones.
                                Proverbs 17:22

Happiness is a perfume
    you can't pour on others without getting
        a few drops on yourself.
                          Ralph Waldo Emerson

Happiness is a habit. Cultivate it.
                              Elbert Hubbard

Cheerfulness is the best promoter of health
and is as friendly to the mind as to the body.
                              Joseph Addison

He who sings frightens
away his ills.

Miguel de Cervantes

The best of healers
is good cheer.

Pindar

Strengthen yourself with contentment,
for it is an impregnable fortress.

Epictetus

He whose face gives no light
shall never be a star.

William Blake

Be. Live. And don't worry too much
about the troubles that loom so large today.
They will pass.

Mickey Rooney

Happiness must be, for most people, an
achievement rather than a gift from the gods.

Bertrand Russell

The art of living lies less in eliminating
our troubles than in growing with them.

Bernard Baruch

The growth of wisdom may be gauged
accurately by the decline of ill temper.

Friedrich Nietzsche

Attitudes, beliefs, and emotional states
ranging from love and compassion to fear and
anger can trigger chain reactions that affect
blood chemistry, heart rate, and the activity
of every cell and organ system in the body.

Kenneth R. Pelletier, Ph.D.

Anger tortures itself.

Publilius Syrus

A grateful mind is a great mind which
eventually attracts to itself great things.

Plato

A thankful heart is not only the greatest
virtue but the parent of all other virtues.

Cicero

The best way to cheer yourself up
is to try to cheer somebody else up.

Mark Twain

Think as little as possible about yourself
and as much as possible about other people.

Eleanor Roosevelt

Scatter seeds of kindness.

George Ade

A loving heart is the truest wisdom.

Charles Dickens

Be kind, for everyone you meet is fighting
a hard battle.

Plato

So it is of cheerfulness:
The more it is spent,
the more of it remains.

Ralph Waldo Emerson

A cloudy day is no match
for a sunny disposition.

William Arthur Ward

If you love life, life will love you back.

Artur Rubinstein

Each day provides its own gifts.

Martial

Thoughts have the power of making us
profoundly happy even while our body
is suffering.

John Cowper Powys

You feel the way you think.

Albert Ellis

A good disposition is a virtue in itself,
and it is lasting.

Ovid

There is overwhelming evidence
that unhealthy motivations can, in certain
situations, produce the chronic emotional
imbalances that predispose us to illness.

Howard S. Friedman, Ph.D.

The best part of health is a fine disposition.

Ralph Waldo Emerson

There ain't much fun in medicine, but there's
a heck of a lot of medicine in fun.

Josh Billings

Rest and be thankful.

William Wordsworth

Happiness is a matter of your own doing. You can be happy or you can be unhappy. It's just according to the way you look at things.

Walt Disney

Talk happiness. The world is sad enough without your woe.

Ella Wheeler Wilcox

Though misfortune may make a man unhappy, she can never make him completely and inseparably miserable without his own consent.

The Old Farmer's Almanac, 1800

The greater part of our happiness depends on our disposition and not our circumstances.

Martha Washington

We must will to be happy, and work at it.

Alain

The mind is like a clock
that is constantly
running down. It has
to be wound up daily
with good thoughts.

Bishop Fulton J. Sheen

This is the day which the Lord hath made; we will rejoice and be glad in it.

Psalms 118:24

Exercise, laughter and play are all closely
related. All three produce similar effects
on the body and mind.

Bernie Siegel, M.D.

Laugh and the world laughs with you.
Weep and you weep alone.

Ella Wheeler Wilcox

Of all the gifts bestowed on human beings,
hearty laughter must be close to the top.

Norman Cousins

Humor makes all things tolerable.

Henry Ward Beecher

Never miss a chance to laugh out loud.

Douglas Fairbanks, Jr.

3

Faith

G. K. Chesterton wrote, "There is one thing which gives radiance to everything. It is the idea of something around the corner." But during periods of ill health, we're hesitant to look around the corner for fear of what we might find. As Paul Valéry observed, "We hope vaguely but dread precisely."

Faith is a powerful tool for the restoration of health. Your body is working overtime to heal itself; you make its job easier if you never stop believing that recovery is at hand. This belief will give radiance to everything as it hastens the healing process.

On the following pages, you will explore the healing power of mountain-moving faith. These quotations will encourage you to hope precisely. And that's precisely what's called for.

Faith is the antiseptic of the soul.

Walt Whitman

Nothing in life is more wonderful than faith
— the one great moving force which
we can neither weigh in the balance
nor test in the crucible.

Sir William Osler

Confidence, deep purpose, joyousness,
laughter, and the will to live increase the
value of the medical treatment we receive.

Norman Cousins

The care of tuberculosis depends more
on what the patient has in his head than
what he has in his chest.

Sir William Osler

Faith is an activity; it is something that has
to be applied.

Corrie Ten Boom

Faith is not believing that God can,
but that God will!

Abraham Lincoln

Faith can put a candle in the darkest night.

Margaret Sangster

He does not believe who does not live
according to his beliefs.

Thomas Fuller

It is part of the cure to wish to be cured.

Seneca

Worry and anxiety are sand
   in the machinery of life; faith is the oil.

E. Stanley Jones

In adversity, a man is saved by hope.

Menander

They can conquer who believe they can.

Ralph Waldo Emerson

Faith is the force of life.

Leo Tolstoy

Beliefs shape the power
of the treatment as well
as the seriousness
of the side effects.

Bernie Siegel, M.D.

Faith is kept alive in us, and gathers strength, more from practice than from speculations.

Joseph Addison

Faith is not belief without proof, but trust without reservations.

Elton Trueblood

Nothing is impossible to a willing heart.

John Heywood

Begin to weave, and God will give the thread.

German Proverb

Alas! The fearful unbelief is unbelief
          in yourself.

Thomas Carlyle

Fear knocked at the door. Faith answered.
          No one was there.

Inscription, Hind's Head Inn, Bray, England

True faith is never found alone;
          it is accompanied by expectation.

C. S. Lewis

Daughter, thy faith hath made thee whole.

Jesus (Mark 5:34)

To me, faith means not worrying.

John Dewey

Some men storm imaginary Alps all their lives and die in the foothills cursing difficulties which do not exist.

Edgar Watson Howe

Live in day-tight compartments.

Dale Carnegie

Great hope makes great men.

Thomas Fuller

There are paths of possibility, towards
which it is also our duty to hold aloft the light,
and the name of that light is hope.

Karl Menninger

Never take away hope from any human being.

Oliver Wendell Holmes, Sr.

I'm not sure anyone knows enough
to deny hope.

Norman Cousins

Honor the healing power of nature.

Hippocrates

4
Patience

Of course you are anxious to feel better, but don't be impatient. Healing takes time. Despite great advances in medicine, the biggest part of your recovery is attributable to the enormous healing power inside you. The body heals itself according to its own timetable — anxious thoughts never hasten recuperation.

Honoré de Balzac noted, "All human power is a compound of time and patience." If you are dissatisfied with the pace of your recovery, calm down. Be a patient patient. Your body is working as fast as it can, so let it work in peace.

The best cure for the body is to quiet the mind.

Napoleon I

Never think that God's delays are God's denials.

Buffon

The principal part of faith is patience.

George Macdonald

Patience means waiting without anxiety.

Saint Francis of Sales

Prayer is not getting, but becoming.

Sidney Greenberg

Waiting patiently in expectation
is the foundation of the spiritual life.

Simone Weil

Patience is power; with time and patience
the mulberry leaf becomes silk.

Chinese Proverb

He who labors diligently need never despair;
for all things are accomplished by diligence
and labor.

Menander

We do not meet with success except
by reiterated efforts.

Françoise de Maintenon

Patience and diligence, like faith,
move mountains.

William Penn

Genius is nothing but a greater aptitude
for patience.

Ben Franklin

The secret of success is constancy of purpose.

Benjamin Disraeli

Little strokes fell great oaks.

Poor Richard's Almanac

Victory belongs to the most persevering.

Napoleon I

Patience is a bitter plant but it has sweet fruit.

German Proverb

Bring forth fruit with patience.

Luke 8:15

The greatest prayer is patience.

Buddha

Trust God to weave your thread
into the great web, though the pattern
shows it not yet.

George Macdonald

To know how to wait is the great secret
to success.

de Maistre

Patient waiting is often the highest way
of doing God's will.

Collier

There is no great achievement that is not
the result of patient working and waiting.

J. G. Holland

There is as much
difference between
genuine patience and
sullen endurance
as between the smile of
love and the malicious
gnashing of teeth.

W. S. Plummer

There is nothing so bitter that a patient
mind cannot find some solace in it.

Seneca

Patience and time do more than strength
or passion.

La Fontaine

To do nothing is sometimes a good remedy.

Hippocrates

He conquers who endures.

Persius

5

Optimism

A little optimism never hurts anyone; to the contrary, sometimes it helps. In his book *Learned Optimism*, Dr. Martin Seligman wrote, "Laboratories around the world have produced a steady flow of scientific evidence that psychological traits, particularly optimism, can produce good health." These words point out an important truth: The self-fulfilling prophecy is alive, well, and working overtime in the field of medicine.

Shakespeare observed, "'Tis the mind that makes the body rich." It's time to enrich *your* body with a healthy dose of optimistic thinking. After all, it can't hurt. Besides, optimists have more fun — or at least they think they do.

Now there is good evidence that this sort
of optimism can improve the quality of a
person's life — and more. It can also play a
key role in maintaining physical health.

Christopher Peterson, M.D. and Lisa M. Bossio

Say you are well, or all is well with you,
and God shall hear your words
and make them true.

Ella Wheeler Wilcox

If a person can turn from predicting illness
to anticipating recovery, the foundation
for cure is laid.

Bernie Siegel, M.D.

Mind and body are
inextricably linked, and
their second-by-second
interaction exerts a
profound influence upon
health and illness,
life and death.

Kenneth R. Pelletier, Ph.D.

Patients tend to move
along the path of their
expectations, whether
on the upside or
the downside.

Norman Cousins

A sad soul can kill you quicker than a germ.

John Steinbeck

Despair is an evil counselor.

Sir Walter Scott

Pray not for crutches, but for wings.

Phillips Brooks

No life is so hard that you can't make
it easier by the way you take it.

Ellen Glasgow

Think of all the ills from which you are exempt.

Joseph Joubert

Never cease to be convinced that life
might be better — your own and others.

André Gide

Gladly accept the gifts of the present hour.

Horace

If I believe there is nothing I can do,
then I can do nothing.

Alain

Do not borrow trouble by dreading tomorrow.
It is the dark menace of the future
that makes cowards of us all.

Dorothy Dix

Worry is interest paid on trouble
before it falls due.

William Ralph Inge

Happiness doesn't depend upon who you are
or what you have; it depends upon
what you think.

Dale Carnegie

Hope is a much greater stimulant of life
than any happiness.

Friedrich Nietzsche

All human wisdom is summed up
in two words — wait and hope.

Alexandre Dumas

The clearest sign of wisdom
is continued cheerfulness.

Michel de Montaigne

He that is of a merry heart
hath a continual feast.

Proverbs 15:15

So great a power is there of the soul upon the body, that whichever way the soul imagines and dreams that it goes, so it leads the body.

Agrippa, 1510

At the core of pessimism is another phenomenon — that of helplessness.

Martin Seligman, Ph.D.

In the long run, the pessimist may be proved to be right, but the optimist has a better time on the trip.

Daniel L. Reardon

I am an optimist. It does not seem too much use being anything else.

Sir Winston Churchill

Optimism is the faith that leads
to achievement. Nothing can be done without
hope and confidence.

Helen Keller

A pessimist is one who makes difficulties
of his opportunities. An optimist is one who
makes opportunities of his difficulties.

Harry S. Truman

The pessimist sees the difficulty in every
opportunity; the optimist sees
the opportunity in every difficulty.

Lawrence Pearsall Jacks

It doesn't hurt to be optimistic.
You can always cry later.

Lucimar Santos de Lima

Unexpected healing happens often enough
that physicians must learn to project hope
at all times.

Bernie Siegel, M.D.

Dear Lord, never let me be afraid to pray
for the impossible.

Dorothy Shellenberger

One of the most effective ways to neutralize
medical pessimism is to find someone
who had the same problem you do
and is now healed.

Andrew Weil, M.D.

There are no incurable diseases.

Bernie Siegel, M.D.

Live from miracle to miracle.

Artur Rubinstein

Whan a man is willing and eager,
the gods join in.

Aeschylus

Man is what he believes.

Anton Chekhov

They are able who think they are able.

Virgil

The greatest discovery of my generation
is that a human being can alter his life
by altering the attitude of his mind.

William James

We see things as we are, not as they are.

Leo Rosten

Human thoughts have the tendency to turn themselves into their physical equivalents.

Earl Nightingale

Drugs are not always
necessary. Belief in
recovery always is.

Norman Cousins

6

Courage

2500 years ago, the Greek dramatist Euripides wrote, "This is courage in a man: To bear unflinchingly what heaven sends."

Obviously, Euripides never saw a hypodermic needle. When heaven sends sickness — or when doctors point needles — it's hard not to flinch.

If you're in the sick bed, you already know that ill health is no place for sissies. So flinch if you must, but do the courageous thing anyway … and get it over with.

Hold positive images and goals in your
mind, pictures of what you truly want in your
life. When fearful images arise, refocus on
images that evoke feelings of peace and joy.

Bernie Siegel, M.D.

Courage is the price life extracts
for granting peace.

Amelia Earhart

What a new face courage puts on everything.

Ralph Waldo Emerson

The first and great commandment
is don't let them scare you.

Elmer Davis

Do not pray for tasks equal to your powers.
Pray for powers equal to your task.

Phillips Brooks

Pray not for safety from danger,
but for deliverance from fear.

Ralph Waldo Emerson

God allows us to experience the low points
of life in order to teach us lessons
we could learn in no other way.

C. S. Lewis

I love the man that can smile in trouble,
that can gather strength from distress and
grow brave by reflection.

Thomas Paine

Men see clearer in times of adversity.
Storms purify the atmosphere.

Henry Ward Beecher

Bad times have a scientific value. These are
occasions a good learner would not miss.

Ralph Waldo Emerson

Difficulties are God's errands and trainers,
and only through them can one come to
the fullness of humanity.

Henry Ward Beecher

Ask yourself, "What's the worst that can happen?" Prepare to accept it. Then improve upon the worst.

Dale Carnegie

Our greatest foes, and whom we chiefly
combat, are within.

Miguel de Cervantes

Courage conquers all things.

Ovid

The desire for safety stands against
every great and noble experience.

Tacitus

When in doubt, do the courageous thing.

Jan Smuts

The only security is courage.

La Rochefoucauld

Never take counsel of your fears.

Andrew Jackson

Life shrinks or expands in proportion
to one's courage.

Anaïs Nin

You cannot run away from a weakness;
you must sometimes fight it out or perish.
And if that be so, why not now,
and from where you stand?

Robert Louis Stevenson

I would define true courage to be a perfect
sensibility of the measure of danger
and a mental willingness to endure it.
General William Tecumseh Sherman

C ourage is resistance to fear, mastery
of fear, not absence of fear.
Mark Twain

W hen pain is to be borne, a little courage
helps more than much knowledge.
C. S. Lewis

I t takes courage to be happy.
Mark Van Doren

Our strength often increases in proportion
to the obstacles imposed upon it.

Rapin

Know how sublime a thing it is to suffer
and be strong.

Henry Wadsworth Longfellow

God will not look you over for medals,
degrees or diplomas, but for scars.

Elbert Hubbard

The greater the difficulty, the more glory
in surmounting it.

Epictetus

Courage can achieve everything.

Sam Houston

Courage is always safer than cowardice.

Old-Time Saying

What does not destroy me
makes me stronger.

Friedrich Nietzsche

You gain strength, courage and confidence
by every experience in which you really stop
to look fear in the face. You must do the thing
you think you cannot do.

Eleanor Roosevelt

Become so wrapped up in something
that you forget to be afraid.

Lady Bird Johnson

Nothing is more valuable to a man than courage.

Terence

Happiness is a form of courage.

Holbrook Jackson

Medical research is discovering that high
determination and purpose can actually
enhance the working of the immune system.

Norman Cousins

To unblock the fountain of love and enter on
the path of creative, spiritual growth,
we must let go of our fears.

Bernie Siegel, M.D.

Keep your fears to yourself, but share your courage.

Robert Louis Stevenson

Have courage for the great sorrows of life and patience for the small ones; and when you have laboriously accomplished your daily task, go to sleep in peace.
God is awake.

Victor Hugo

7

Acceptance

Acceptance is paradoxical. Sometimes, we must accept things *before* we can change them. This is especially true in the treatment of serious illness. Bernie Siegel, M.D. wrote, "A serene acceptance of *what is* promotes health, but by keeping the mind clear it also puts a person in a better position to change things that need changing."

Accepting your illness doesn't mean giving in to it. Acceptance is simply a first step in the healing process. Then, once you've accepted "what is," you are free to begin working on "what will be."

There is only one way to happiness and that is to cease worrying about things that are beyond the power of our will.

Epictetus

Acceptance, submission, surrender —
whatever one chooses to call it, this mental
shift may be the master key
that unlocks healing.

Andrew Weil, M.D.

Know when to let your doctor take over.
There's nothing to be gained by obsessing
about situations you can't control. When things
are out of your hands, the best advice is to stay
relaxed and hope for the best.

Tom Ferguson, M.D.

If you haven't the strength to impose
your own terms upon life, you must accept
the terms it offers you.

T. S. Eliot

Bear, do not blame, what cannot be changed.

Publilius Syrus

Self-pity is our worst enemy. If we yield to it,
we can never do anything wise in the world.

Helen Keller

Blessed are those who forget, for they thus
surmount even their own mistakes.

Friedrich Nietzsche

Guilt about illness is destructive; it cannot
possibly help the healing system.

Andrew Weil, M.D.

God asks no man whether he will accept life.
That is not the choice. You *must* take it.
The only choice is *how*.

Henry Ward Beecher

Strengthen yourself with contentment,
for it is an impregnable fortress.

Epictetus

In His will is our peace.

Dante

True peace is found by man in the depths
of his own heart, the dwelling place of God.

Johannes Tauler

The man who has become emancipated
from the empire of worry will find life a much
more cheerful affair than it used to be while
he was perpetually being irritated.

Bertrand Russell

Accept things as they are,
not as you wish them to be.

Napoleon I

Prudence dictates to us to make the best
we can of inevitable evils. We may fret and
fume and peeve and scold and rave,
but what good will it do us?

John Adams

Change seems more likely to occur in a
climate of surrender than in a climate
of confrontation with the universe.

Andrew Weil, M.D.

Ask not that events happen as they will,
but let your will be that events happen as
they do, and you shall have peace.

Epictetus

There is nothing the body suffers that the soul may not profit by.

George Meredith

Every man's life is a plan of God.

Horace Bushnell

As in a game of cards, so in the game of life
we must play what is dealt to us; and the
glory consists not so much in winning,
as in playing a poor hand well.

Josh Billings

Release all negative emotions —
resentment, envy, fear, sadness, anger.
Express your feelings appropriately; don't
hold on to them. And forgive yourself.

Bernie Siegel, M.D.

Life does not have to be
perfect to be wonderful.

Annette Funicello

For what has been —
thanks.
For what shall be —
yes!

Dag Hammarskjöld

God grant me the serenity
to accept the things
I cannot change;
the courage to change
the things I can;
and the wisdom to know
the difference.

Reinhold Niebuhr

8

Healthy Living

Thomas Edison predicted, "The doctor of the future will give no medicine but will interest his patients in the care of the human frame and in the cause and prevention of disease." He was partially correct. Despite Edison's prediction to the contrary, physicians still give medication. But on another level, Edison was a visionary. Although medicine plays an ever-increasing role in the treatment of disease, so does prevention. Our job, whether healthy or otherwise, is to head off sickness at the pass. We do so when we adopt healthy habits.

Dr. Samuel Johnson observed, "The chains of habit are too weak to be felt until they are too strong to be broken." If you are enchained by bad habits, fashion your escape today.

True enjoyment comes from activity of the mind and exercise of the body: the two are ever united.

Baron Alexander von Humboldt

Walking is man's best medicine.

Hippocrates

It is impossible to walk rapidly
and be unhappy.

Howard Murphy, M.D.

To ward off disease or recover health,
man as a rule finds it easier to depend on
healers than to attempt the more difficult task
of living wisely.

René Dubos

Make a commitment to health and well
being, and develop a belief in the possibility
of total health. Develop your own healing
program, drawing on the support and advice
of experts without becoming enslaved
to them.

Bernie Siegel, M.D.

The best health care combines self care
with professional advice.

Tom Ferguson, M.D.

Stopping an illness before it begins
is known as preventative medicine.
It is the medicine of the future.
Mike Samuels, M.D. and Nancy Samuels

Attention to one's lifestyle, especially in the
direction of reducing emotional tensions,
a modest but regular program of daily exercise,
a diet low in salt and sugar and reasonably free
of fatty meats and fried foods, and plenty of
good drinking water — all these are useful and
indeed essential.
Norman Cousins

Disease can be a motivator for change.

Bernie Siegel, M.D.

The challenge is to use sickness
as an opportunity for transformation.

Andrew Weil, M.D.

Changing behaviors accomplishes little
if we do not change how we think.

Paul Pearsall, M.D.

Exercise and physical fitness can act
as buffers against stress.

Michael H. Sacks, M.D.

Exercisers tend to be less depressed
than people who don't exercise.
That much is known.

Michael H. Sacks, M.D.

People who exercise regularly
have fewer illnesses.

Bernie Siegel, M.D.

We never repent of having eaten too little.
Thomas Jefferson

Eat to live and not live to eat.
Poor Richard's Almanac

Don't mistake pleasure for happiness.
Josh Billings

Everything in excess is opposed to nature.

Hippocrates

Health is not simply the absence of illness.

Hannah Green

The *body* heals, not the therapy.

Bernie Siegel, M.D.

We are spinning our own fates, good or evil,
and never to be undone.

William James

The physician is only nature's assistant.

Galen

9

Treasure Each Day

When we're under the weather, it's easy to lose count of our blessings. But even sick days are gifts from above, not to be taken for granted. Jonathan Swift anticipated the challenge of the daily grind when he penned this simple benediction: "May you live all the days of your life." Presumably, Swift meant *all* days, not just the days when we feel our best.

Each new dawn brings its own special bundle of opportunities. Today is a blessing of God. We should use this blessing wisely, enjoy it, and give thanks. Swiftly.

Do not act as if you had a thousand years to live.

Marcus Aurelius

Begin at once to live, and count each day as a separate life.

Seneca

Doth thou love life?
Then do not squander time, for that's
the stuff life is made of.

Ben Franklin

Tomorrow's life is too late. Live today.

Martial

Plunge boldly into the thick of life!

Goethe

Live now, believe me, wait not till tomorrow;
gather the roses of life today.

Pierre de Ronsard

Nobody's gonna live for you.

Dolly Parton

Time is really the only capital that any
human being has and the only thing
he can't afford to lose.

Thomas Edison

The passing minute is every man's
equal possession.

Marcus Aurelius

Brief is the space of life allotted to you;
pass it as pleasantly as you can, not grieving
from noon till eve.

Euripides

Every man's life lies within the present, for
the past is spent and the future is uncertain.

Marcus Antonius

One today is worth two tomorrows.

Ben Franklin

Life is a journey,
not a destination.
Happiness is not "there",
but here, not tomorrow,
but today.

Sidney Greenberg

Find the journey's end in every step.

Ralph Waldo Emerson

Hope of gain lessens pain.

Poor Richard's Almanac

He who fears he shall suffer, already suffers
what he fears.

Michel de Montaigne

Each of us makes his own weather,
determines the color of the skies in the
emotional universe which he inhabits.

Bishop Fulton J. Sheen

Man is what he believes.

Anton Chekhov

Life begins on the other side of despair.

Jean-Paul Sartre

Follow your desire
as long as you live;
do not lessen the time
of following desire,
for the wasting of time
is an abomination
to the spirit.

Ptahhotep, 2350 BC

A happy life is one
that is in accordance
with its own nature.

Seneca

Plenty of people miss their share of happiness, not because they never found it, but because they didn't stop to enjoy it.

William Feather

There is more to life than increasing its speed.

Mohandas Gandhi

Is life so wretched? Isn't it rather your hands which are too small, your vision which is muddled? You are the one who must grow up.

Dag Hammarskjöld

We fear our highest possibilities. We are generally afraid to become that which we can glimpse in our most perfect moments, under the most perfect conditions, under conditions of great courage.

Abraham Maslow

Write on your heart that every day
is the best day of the year.
Ralph Waldo Emerson

Life is what we make it. Always has been.
Always will be.
Grandma Moses

Life is really simple, but men insist on
making it complicated.
Confucius

We find in life exactly what we put in.
Ralph Waldo Emerson

Live so that you were not born in vain.

Cicero

Do not walk through time without leaving worthy evidence of your passage.

Pope John XXIII

Live out your life in its full meaning.
It is God's life.

Josiah Royce

We are citizens of eternity.

Dostoyevsky

Never run out of goals.

Earl Nightingale

The greatest use of life is to spend it
for something that will outlast it.

William James

This is happiness; to be dissolved
into something complete and great.

Willa Cather

Life is either a daring adventure or nothing.

Helen Keller

The right time is any time that one is still
so lucky as to have. Live!

Henry James

The tragedy of life is not so much what men suffer but what they miss.

Thomas Carlyle

Make your life a mission — not an intermission.

Arnold Glasow

Life is not breath, but action.
    Life consists less in length of days
    than in the keen sense of living.
            Jean-Jacques Rousseau

It is not death that a man should fear,
    but he should fear never beginning to live.
            Marcus Aurelius

A long life may not be good enough,
    but a good life is long enough.
            Poor Richard's Almanac

Do not take life too seriously.
    You'll never get out of it alive.
            Elbert Hubbard

<u>10</u>

All-Purpose Advice

We conclude with a few observations about doctors, patients, visiting hours and other facts of medical life. Enjoy.

Pick a doctor you like
before there is
an emergency.

Tom Ferguson, M.D.

God cures and the doctor sends the bill.

Mark Twain

Life can only be understood backwards;
    but it must be lived forwards.

Søren Kierkegaard

We cannot learn without pain.

Aristotle

He knows not his own strength
    that hath not met adversity.

Ben Jonson

There is no education like adversity.

Benjamin Disraeli

Perhaps perseverance has been the radical
principle of every truly great character.

John Foster

The greater the obstacle, the more glory
in overcoming it.

Molière

The saints are sinners who keep on going.

Robert Louis Stevenson

When life kicks you, let it kick you forward.

E. Stanley Jones

Healing proceeds from the depths
to the heights.

Carl Jung

The healing path is made up of the steps we
take to enact our own potential — steps that
may lead into every region of our lives.

Marc Ian Barasch

God helps the sick in two ways: through the
science of medicine and surgery, and through
the science of faith and prayer.

Norman Vincent Peale

The human body is far more robust
than people have been led to believe.

Norman Cousins

The body wants to be healthy.
This is the natural condition. When the body
is out of balance, it wants to get back to it.

Andrew Weil, M.D.

Natural forces within us are
the true healers of disease.

Hippocrates

Choose a doctor who shares your personal
style and philosophy.

Tom Ferguson, M.D.

Full communication between patient
and physician is indispensable for accurate
diagnosis and effective treatment.

Norman Cousins

No one is wise enough by himself.

Titus Maccius Plautus

Let great physicians cure the dangerous ills.

Juvenal

You are in charge of setting your own visiting
hours. Take charge of your visitors
and ask them to come at the times
that are convenient to you.

Tom Ferguson, M.D.

Arrange visits and calls from those
who will nurture and love you.

Bernie Siegel, M.D.

The pain of the mind is worse
than the pain of the body.

Publilius Syrus

Hostile, depressed, and apathetic people
tend to engage in activities that damage
their health.

Howard S. Friedman, Ph.D.

The surest way to intensify an illness
is to blame oneself or the Deity.

Norman Cousins

Viewing disease as a sign of personal
inadequacy or culpability is both
cruel and false.

Bernie Siegel, M.D.

Have patience with all things,
but first of all with yourself.

Saint Francis of Sales

Happiness is fundamentally a state of mind — not a state of body.

Douglas Fairbanks, Jr.

Pay close and loving attention to yourself,
tuning in to your needs on all levels.
Take care of yourself, nourishing,
supporting and encouraging yourself.

Bernie Siegel, M.D.

The best depression-blockers are
a strong will to live, blazing determination,
and a sense of purpose.

Norman Cousins

Whatever invisible enemies I might swallow
with each mouthful of food, they cannot affect
my heart or stomach any more drastically
than the changes in my moods and
the fantasies of my imagination.

Alain

I have the conviction that when physiology
will be far enough advanced, the poet,
the philosopher and the physiologist
will all understand each other.

Claude Bernard

Troubles are often the tools by which God
fashions us for better things.

Henry Ward Beecher

Sleep, riches and health, to be truly enjoyed,
must be interrupted.

Jean Paul Richter

The world breaks everyone and afterward
many are strong at the broken places.

Ernest Hemingway

As it is not proper to cure the eyes
without the head, nor the head without
the body, so neither is it proper to cure
the body without the soul.

Socrates

Doctors don't know everything, really.
They understand matter, not spirit.
And you and I live in the spirit.

William Saroyan

Love is an element which
binds and heals, which
comforts and restores,
which works what we
must call — for now —
miracles.

Karl Menninger

Sources

Sources

Sources

About the Author

Criswell Freeman is a Doctor of Clinical Psychology living in Nashville, Tennessee. He is the author of *When Life Throws You a Curveball, Hit It* and numerous books in the Wisdom Series published by WALNUT GROVE PRESS.

Dr. Freeman's Wisdom Books chronicle memorable quotations in an easy-to-read style. The series provides inspiring, thoughtful and humorous messages from entertainers, athletes, scientists, politicians, clerics, writers and renegades, with each title focusing on a particular region or area of special interest. Combining his passion for quotations with extensive training in psychology, Freeman revisits timeless themes such as perseverance, courage, love, forgiveness and faith.

Dr. Freeman is also the host of *Wisdom Made in America*, a nationally syndicated radio program.

The Wisdom Series
by Dr. Criswell Freeman

Regional Titles

Wisdom Made in America	ISBN 1-887655-07-7
The Book of Southern Wisdom	ISBN 0-9640955-3-X
The Wisdom of the Midwest	ISBN 1-887655-17-4
The Wisdom of the West	ISBN 1-887655-31-X
The Book of Texas Wisdom	ISBN 0-9640955-8-0
The Book of Florida Wisdom	ISBN 0-9640955-9-9
The Book of California Wisdom	ISBN 1-887655-14-X
The Book of New York Wisdom	ISBN 1-887655-16-6
The Book of New England Wisdom	ISBN 1-887655-15-8

Sports Titles

The Golfer's Book of Wisdom	ISBN 0-9640955-6-4
The Putter Principle	ISBN 1-887655-39-5
The Golfer's Guide to Life	ISBN 1-887655-38-7
The Wisdom of Women's Golf	ISBN 1-887655-82-4
The Book of Football Wisdom	ISBN 1-887655-18-2
The Wisdom of Southern Football	ISBN 0-9640955-7-2
The Book of Stock Car Wisdom	ISBN 1-887655-12-3
The Wisdom of Old-Time Baseball	ISBN 1-887655-08-5
The Book of Basketball Wisdom	ISBN 1-887655-32-8
The Fisherman's Guide to Life	ISBN 1-887655-30-1
The Tennis Lover's Guide to Life	ISBN 1-887655-36-0

Special People Titles

Mothers Are Forever	ISBN 1-887655-76-X
Fathers Are Forever	ISBN 1-887655-77-8
Friends Are Forever	ISBN 1-887655-78-6
The Teachers' Book of Wisdom	ISBN 1-887655-80-8
The Graduates' Book of Wisdom	ISBN 1-887655-81-6
The Guide to Better Birthdays	ISBN 1-887655-35-2
Get Well Soon…If Not Sooner	ISBN 1-887655-79-4
The Wisdom of the Heart	ISBN 1-887655-34-4

Special Interest Titles

The Book of Country Music Wisdom	ISBN 0-9640955-1-3
Old-Time Country Wisdom	ISBN 1-887655-26-3
The Wisdom of Old-Time Television	ISBN 1-887655-64-6
The Book of Cowboy Wisdom	ISBN 1-887655-41-7
The Gardener's Guide to Life	ISBN 1-887655-40-9
The Salesman's Book of Wisdom	ISBN 1-887655-83-2
Minutes from the Great Women's Coffee Club (by Angela Beasley)	ISBN 1-887655-33-6

Wisdom Books are available at fine stores everywhere.
For information about a retailer near you, call 1-800-256-8584.